Stopping Emotional Eating:

HeartMath® Stress and Weight Management Program

Integrating emWave® and Inner Balance™ Technologies

Doc Childre and Deborah Rozman, Ph.D.
with Sheva Carr

+💜 **HeartMath**.

14700 West Park Avenue
Boulder Creek, CA 95006
800–450-9111
www.heartmath.com

Introduction

In 1991, Doc Childre founded the non-profit Institute of HeartMath and began research into the underlying mechanisms of stress and behavior change. Based on this research, Doc and the HeartMath team developed user-friendly tools and technologies to transform stress and empower behavior change. Users progress through their own reward – you feel better using them and you see results – which builds initiative to transform more stress. You learn to manage emotional reactions and clear emotional undercurrents until you create a new baseline of emotional behavior—a neural habit change.

Note from Doc Childre

Look at this booklet as a friend and a facilitator for whatever weight management process you choose. The intention of this book is not to assess or judge any process, but to help people add more of the core values of the heart to their diet adventures. Connecting more with the heart helps to bring the emotions into balance, which by now most know is a missing piece, a serious "x" factor in weight management. Eating is so strongly connected with our feelings (be they happy, sad, anxious, lonely, overloaded or depressed) that the balance between heart, mind and emotions has to be included in our diet commitments and intentions.

To align with your intuitive heart intelligence is not just for dieting, but a practical way to approach life. The increase in stress, time pressures and information overload these days can make it tough to diet or even "breathe" at times. All of the stress can't be eliminated, but approaching it through the heart can take much significance out of issues that have to be dealt with and can prevent the negative impact of stress before it accumulates. A lot of stress and stress eating can be eliminated as you learn to have compassion for yourself, increase self-acceptance and learn how to say no to "drama." These are some of the key issues that will be addressed in this Program.

"We are putting HeartMath programs directly into the center of our employee health and wellness program in addition to our corporate wellness programs. What we are finding is that if we are able to help people better control the stress in their lives, they actually get more engaged in other healthy behaviors like diet, exercise and tobacco cessation and with better outcomes. For example average per employee cost for conditions related to overweight or obesity is approximately $4300. For employees who participated in our 'I Choose Health' wellness program, the average cost was $82 per employee. We feel that HeartMath's unique science-based approach to stress management is the foundation of preventative health."

—Todd C Linden, CEO, Grinnell Regional Medical Center

Overview

Part 1 of this book covers important basics for stopping emotional eating with key strategies for success.

Part 2 of this book provides step-by-step instructions for the *HeartMath Stress and Weight Management Program* to be followed over the course of six weeks (or longer to suit your needs). You will gain a deeper understanding of how and why this program works along with inspiration and encouragement as you follow the Program. You can learn more about the scientific background behind the HeartMath tools and technologies in the Appendix.

Part 3 of this book is a Quick Start Guide for those of you who want to get started right away. It includes quick start summary pages (tool cheat sheet and daily practice plan).

Acknowledgements

This program has been in development over several years and many people have contributed to its success. We thank them all for their insights into the emotional side of weight management. We thank Ted Barasch for his encouragement and comments based on his many years of experience in the weight loss industry, Charles Inlander and Donna Beech for their editorial contributions, and Barbara Birsinger for her research on intuitive eating. We also thank the *HeartMath Stress and Weight Management* pilot study participants and Institute of HeartMath researchers Jackie Waterman and Mike Atkinson who conducted the pilot study. We especially thank Sheva Carr, program coordinator for the pilot study participants, who significantly contributed to the content of this book.

Stopping Emotional Eating Beta Test Results

A pilot study of 19 participants using the *HeartMath Stress and Weight Management Program* showed the following results in just six weeks:

- There was a significant 5.2 lb reduction in the group average weight.
- Average waist circumference was significantly reduced by 2.1 inches
- Average hip circumference was significantly reduced by 1.78 inches
- Calmness significantly increased
- Anger, resentfulness and stress were all significantly lower at the post study measurement.

Comments from *HeartMath Stress and Weight Management Program* Participants:

"If it hadn't been for the hope this program gave me and measurements that the HeartMath technology provided, I would not be where I am today. I have lost 9 pounds and kept it off since finishing the beta test more than 6 months ago. The bonus is that my health and other aspects of my life have also improved. Losing weight was not as important as controlling the emotional chaos I was experiencing. I feel healthier, more energized and I am sleeping better. I firmly believe I am going to continue to lose weight because I am no longer compulsive eating to handle my issues."

April Mydske, Manager, WA

"This is a GREAT program! You get calm and you lose weight all at the same time!"

Colleen, Administrative Secretary, Fairfield Medical Center, OH

"Just do it and watch the results!"

Jim Kettering, Pilot, School administrator, CO

"Heightened awareness from this program leads to VERY significant behavioral change."

Mina Ubbing, Fairfield Medical Center CEO, OH

"This program has taught me to pay attention, to go inside myself for resources, and having the technology is a physical link to help you actually do that instead of just know that you should."

Julie Hiebert, MN

"I know in my heart that it is because of the HeartMath tools and using the HeartMath technology that I was able to lose 75 lbs. Before practicing HeartMath tools, I had yoyo-ed in my weight, but the most I had ever lost was 15 pounds and then gained it back.

Now, it has been more than 18 months since I started and I have no problem keeping the weight off.

When I decided to take my weight loss really seriously was the day I started practicing HeartMath tools. Before using HeartMath tools, food was what I used as my comfort. Food was always available, was quiet, and did not talk back. When I felt emotionally upset, I would not limit myself in what I ate. And food is socially acceptable. Even other people use it to comfort you and nurture you.

I started to use the HeartMath tools when I felt stress instead of food, which gave me power and freedom inside the gap between cause and effect, between eating and blindly reacting. When I tried to lose weight before using the HeartMath tools, I thought the mountain was too high to climb, I thought, 'I cannot do this.' With HeartMath practice, I could take it one moment at a time, and the tools gave me the winning recipe to feel like I COULD do it. Using the HeartMath technology finally gave me the power to say to myself that this excess food is not good for me, I don't want it. It gave me a security where I could say to myself, 'I can do this'.

I took it one craving at a time, day in and day out. As silly as it sounds, every time I zip up my pants or get down to a smaller size, I use one of my HeartMath skills of appreciation, and I appreciate where I am, what I did, who I am now, how I feel, what people say, the size and the clothes I can now wear, and I just keep feeling appreciation of those things.

HeartMath taught me that appreciation is self love and care and it's healthy for me. All the time, every moment, there are opportunities to incorporate what I learned from HeartMath in to my day to day life.

Now I feel so free. I have a new life. I like myself better, I feel free from the trap of a heavy body. Society is tough on you anyway— you cannot be too thin. So to be successful in weight loss, I needed to find a place inside me that loved me in the face of all the judgments that were around me. HeartMath and the HeartMath technology gave me that.

It's known that 98% of people who lose weight do not keep the weight off. I think that's because they don't do the psychological and emotional part of it too. For me, having HeartMath and the HeartMath technology for the psychological component has been the key to my lasting weight loss success. I really should say thank you HeartMath for the help to get a new life, I am so much happier."

Susan Hanks Marscellas
Vice President, Marketing & Public Relations
Salinas Valley Memorial Healthcare System
Salinas, California

Table of Contents:

Part 1
Stopping Emotional Eating Basics

Stress Eating

Let's face it. We all know that losing weight and keeping it off is hard. That's why there are hundreds of diets available and new diet "solutions" are announced every month. We hope that maybe one of these diets or a new diet pill will do the job, but usually we end up in the same "yo-yo" syndrome. Lose a little, gain it back. Or lose a lot, gain it back. It doesn't have to be that way.

Weight loss specialists and health professionals are realizing that there is a missing "x" factor that most weight management programs have not been addressing adequately. It's called "emotional eating" or "stress eating," and also applies to weight gain related to elevated stress hormones even in the absence of overeating. Once you know how the *missing factor* applies to why you can't manage your weight, you can do something about it. The *HeartMath Stress and Weight Management Program* will give you the tools you need to stop stress eating and to transform your stress into increased balance, peace and creative energy at the same time.

Experts now agree that about 75% of overeating is caused by emotional eating, which means that a lot of us are using food to cope with our feelings. In today's high-stress society, many of us, adults and children, eat high levels of carbohydrate, fat or sugar foods to soothe our emotions or relieve our stress and anxiety. One reason why there's more emotional eating today is that people are crunched for time and under a lot of pressure. In today's fast-paced world, most of us have a lot of loads we carry that add "weight" to our lives. We carry emotional weight, not just physical weight, making it harder to stick to any diet. On top of that, being overweight or being unable to lose weight can be one

1

of the biggest causes of emotional stress in its own right. Weight loss doesn't have to be stressful and that's the hope this program provides.

Maybe you look at yourself in the mirror every morning and announce to yourself, "Today is the day I am going to start losing 50 pounds!" But by midmorning the resolve is gone and you start feeling guilty when you eat that snack, which only causes you to feel helpless, maybe eat more, and get more stressed out.

We understand how challenging it can be to lose weight or to maintain your weight loss. This booklet was written from a deep understanding of human psychology and how the emotional-metabolic system works. It was also written with genuine compassion for the struggle with weight that so many people experience. We will give you new tools you can use to address the missing factor in weight management – the emotions. You will learn how to manage your emotional energies and release your stress - without depending on food to make you feel better.

This may be the only weight management program that doesn't focus on what you eat, but rather on what you feel. You won't see any food lists or exercise regimens in this program. While these are important aspects in reducing weight and improving health, this program focuses on what researchers at the Institute of HeartMath have found to be the first and most important aspect of weight management: regulating your emotions. Learning how to recognize and shift your emotions is a key to success in weight loss and will help other areas of your life as well, including relationships, work, health and quality of life.

You do have the power to achieve and maintain your body's "best weight" goal, but you can't only consider your food diet. In order to achieve and maintain your best weight it's important to address your *emotional diet* as part of a "wholeness diet." It's your attitudes, feelings, self-image, sense of despair and so on—that most determine your ability to stay with a diet plan and not revert to old eating habits.

To help you learn *how* to change your emotional diet, we created the *HeartMath Stress and Weight Management Program*. The Program focuses on the use of key HeartMath tools and the HeartMath technology. The HeartMath tools have been proven in hospitals and clinics to not only reduce stress and increase vitality, but to improve your ability to self-regulate and self-empower behavior change. The HeartMath technology helps train you to shift from stressful feelings to a balanced and dynamic emotional state called *coherence*. Coherence generates an alignment of heart, mind, body and spirit that gives you more power—heart power—to achieve the results you want. The HeartMath technology was developed from over 2 decades of scientific research on the heart, brain and nervous system, conducted by Doc Childre and the Institute of HeartMath. Combining HeartMath tools with HeartMath technology progressively builds the heart power and heart intelligence (a combination of positive emotion and practical intuition) needed to stop emotional eating and maintain your commitments. You learn to eliminate self-defeating energy drains, build the strength to abandon old habits and get back on your feet fast if you do go back to old habits.

Heart power is different from will power.

Will power is a mental activity. It can give you a little momentum, but then it fizzles if there isn't enough heart and emotional commitment behind it. This is because your heart brings in the intuitive intelligence and power of your spirit, which is stronger than just trying to discipline your habits from the mind and will power.

By learning to access this untapped power that lies within your heart, which is the basis of the *HeartMath Stress and Weight*

Management Program, you can reroute your emotions into more beneficial outcomes. Research has shown that the heart sends powerful signals to the brain and rest of the body. Once understood and accessed, these heart signals give you more ability to self-regulate your emotions and nervous system and to make changes you thought you couldn't make before. Throughout history, people have talked about the core values of the heart, which include love, care, appreciation, respect, compassion, kindness, forgiveness and non-judgment. These values and attitudes, which we call core heart feelings, generate the heart signals that bring more coherence to the body's systems. When your initial effort is "from the heart," it brings your mind and emotions into cooperative alignment, and this gives you more intuitive clarity to clear disturbances, and more strength and energy to achieve your goals. That's why coaches say, "play from the heart" or "sing from the heart" or "put your heart into it." Putting your heart into whatever you do gives more power, enjoyment and better results. We'll explain how to do this practically and effectively in this program.

You can use the *HeartMath Stress and Weight Management Program* with *any other weight management or diet program you are using.* You will learn simple steps to release stress in the moment, increase coherence and harness the power of your emotional physiology. As you use the HeartMath tools provided in this program, you will start to feel better and make better choices. You will start to look better and have more energy. We will show you how to use the power and intelligence of your heart intuition to feel better about yourself, your body and your life.

Taming the Inner Critic

If you are like many people struggling with weight, you are probably quite hard on yourself. You may have an inner critic that keeps you stressed with self-judgment and guilt. One of the ways that people try to buffer self-judgment is to eat. They look to food for comfort, and for a temporary physical distraction from the ongoing mental chatter of the inner critic. Of course, after the box of cookies is gone, the inner critic has new ammunition – guilt! And the cycle repeats...

What tends to happen soon after we embark on a weight management program is the heavy-handed inner critic sees a new playground for its self-defeating monologues. "Ha! You're doing this wrong. You aren't using this tool correctly. You are going to fail!" One of the best things about the *HeartMath Stress and Weight Management Program* is that you cannot do this program "wrong." You can drop your measuring sticks or performance anxiety about "did good" or "did bad." Just come back to the present moment and simply use one of the tools you will learn to take care of yourself emotionally right then—whether you "do it right" or not. That's doing the program as intended. Each time you sincerely practice a tool, you are loosening the grip of the inner critic. The tools help you shift into a new attitude toward yourself that will gradually free you of your inner critic and open up new doors of possibility in everything else that you do as well.

Letting Go of "All or Nothing"

Another way that the inner critic emotionally sabotages people is perfectionism. Letting go of trying to be perfect (or giving up when you feel like you're not doing something perfectly) is taking a huge emotional weight off your back. Be kind to yourself as you learn the tools. If you saw a toddler fall down while learning to walk, you wouldn't start berating or judging her. See yourself the same way as you embark on a new relationship with stress and emotions. It's okay to fall. Just get up and try again, the same way you learned to walk.

After eating one piece of cake, people tend to tell themselves, "Well, I've already blown it for today, so I may as well just eat the whole cake and start again tomorrow." That's like a toddler saying, "Well I fell down so I'll just keep crawling and won't try to walk again." Through the tools in this program, you will learn to convert perfectionism and resignation into, "Well, I've eaten one piece of cake and enjoyed it, and that's no big deal. Now I can start again fresh in this moment, right now. I can notice what I was feeling that drove me to eat cake so that I can deal with this emotion right now, rather than stuffing that feeling until it pops up again in another eating binge." That's heart intelligence.

Realize that learning these tools is an adventure between you and your own heart. It is the inner critic that pulls you out of your feelings and into your head. Come back to what you are feeling instead, and keep making choices that feel good to your heart. Free yourself from "performing" the tools to get them right. Instead, keep your attention in your heart, which is non-judgmental, compassionate and gives latitude in the learning process. Each time you let go of performance concerns, self-judgment or guilt, the energy saved will add to your heart power.

Some days you may feel right on track with using the tools, while other days you may feel that you have "fallen off the wagon." It's natural to have ups and downs in any learning process. Keep an eye on the temptation to give up all together on "off" days. Remember its not "all or nothing." When there is greater resistance to following the program, those are usually the times when there is an opportunity to build more muscle, as in exercise. Bring a sense of humor and a spirit of adventure to the process on "off" days. Do your best not to take the inner critic seriously when it uses "off" days to build a case that you are a failure. Remind yourself that ups and downs are built into any growth process in life. It's how we meet them that counts.

Releasing the habit of emotional eating is a process, not a destination. It is not something that you can do cold turkey. Results layer in little by little with new awareness, in increasing ratios of growth and continuity, until one morning you may wake up, like those who have used the HeartMath tools before you, to discover that your habits are changing. Eating emotionally no longer owns you. Just take it a moment at a time, and renew your commitment each day. If you do that, you will be creating a new habit in your relationship to your emotions and food.

It can help to know that if you make a sincere effort to follow this program at the beginning, it will get easier and easier. Researchers at NASA determined that it only takes 21–42 days (3–6 weeks) to create a new habit pattern. In the first three weeks of this program, if you make a sincere effort to practice the tools provided, even if it feels like you are pedaling uphill at times, you can know that the rest of the program can get easier. The 80/20 rule states that 80% of the effort at the beginning yields only 20% of the results. At a certain point there is an inversion and you get 80% of the results for 20% of the effort. In other words, give yourself the gift of knowing that if you continually renew your commitment for just 21 days, you've made it through the hardest phase. You are rewiring a neural habit and using the heart tools to address emotions, and eventually that will become second nature. The benefits will reinforce your new habits in an upward-spiral, as long as you don't let yourself fall into the trap of giving up and rolling all the way down the hill when you slip. Just pick yourself back up when you fall, and renew your commitment here and now. Each time you do this, it counts towards changing your neural habits! You never know which choice will be your tipping point of change.

Making the Tools A Habit: The Heart as Your Default Setting

One of the challenges with changing emotional habits is that the rational part of your brain that learns new tools gets hijacked by the emotions in a stress reaction. It can be frustrating when you have all the best intentions to make new choices and are continually hijacked by old patterns. It is important to have compassion and understanding for the fact that it is natural to default to old habits, especially under stress, and hard for your body, mind and emotions to adopt a new approach as the default setting right away. The key to making a lasting shift and a neural habit change is to apply your tools outside of a stressful context, as in your Quick Start daily practice plan, either in the morning before your day begins or at night when things have quieted down before you go to bed. If you practice the tools in a more controlled environment, they will become second nature after a time, even in the midst of daily stresses. As one participant in the program told us, she dreamed she was in a bank robbery and was teaching the bank teller hiding behind the counter how to breathe through the heart in her dream! Don't expect this "unconscious competence" right away. Just like driving a car, you will need to think about using your tools for a while, but if you commit to doing them daily by the end of your program they will become second nature, as your default response to life.

Boredom and Loneliness

People rarely think of boredom or loneliness as forms of "stress," but they affect heart rhythms and metabolism in much the same way that anxiety, depression and tension do. When we beta-tested this weight management program, we found that boredom and loneliness were two of the most common causes of emotional eating. Both are emotions which people don't often consider to be emotions. They also cover up or "numb" other underlying feelings. Be aware of boredom and loneliness as you track your deficit or draining experiences each day, and apply the tools you are learning to see what the boredom or loneliness may be numbing. Loneliness is often a sign of a lack of heart connection with one's own self. This program will help you re-establish that heart connection. You will learn how you can work with any emotion or attitude that arises within you, neutralize its charge, and harness its energy to create new positive experiences in your life. You will find boredom and loneliness decrease along with the desire to eat emotionally. In the beginning, look at boredom and loneliness as flags pointing you in the right direction of untapped information about yourself and your emotional eating patterns.

Overcoming Insomnia

Many people who struggle with emotional eating fall into the pattern of eating late at night (this is often when people feel lonely or bored). It is common for people under high levels of stress to have reduced serotonin (a neurotransmitter that plays a role in sleep) and to crave carbohydrates before bed as a way to facilitate relaxation and winding down by increasing their serotonin level with food. The HeartMath technology is a wonderful way, calorie free, to help reduce stress hormones, balance the nervous system, increase precursors to serotonin, and wind down without overeating.

(If you are among the many people who struggle with late night eating due to insomnia, you may also want to read *The HeartMath Solution to Better Sleep* e-book.)

Exercise

Often when experiencing anxiety and emotional pain, we don't have the initiative to exercise. However, exercise not only can help to increase your metabolism but also to spin off and clear mental fog and tension accumulated from anxiety, anger and worry. Exercise won't take away your reasons for getting stressed, but it strengthens your capacity to manage your stress with less energy loss, and burns calories to boot. You don't have to do a total workout to help clear your thinking and stabilize your emotions. Experiment and find what's comfortable for you, but at least try to get your heart rate up a little for a period of time. Try to be conscious not to replay negative mind loops while exercising. It helps to balance the emotions and calm the mind if you practice some of the techniques you learn in this book while exercising. Many who have been through this program find that they naturally gravitate to exercise the more they do heart-focused breathing, and that exercise is easier to make a part of their routine with less resistance. If you stop a binge by exercising first, sometimes you can clear the emotional boredom or stress driving you to eat and gain release from exercise instead. Even if you still want to eat after you've excercised, you've burned some of the emotional energy and the calories in advance!

Appreciate Yourself: The Most Valuable Investment You can Make

It is essential to take time to appreciate yourself and your progress every day. Just as stocks which appreciate go up in value, appreciating the progress you make and the qualities you value in yourself adds energy to accomplish more. It makes the process of emotional management more fun too. Appreciating yourself is a very effective antidote to perfectionism and the inner critic. It also helps you overcome the pitfall that many face of longing to have the body they once had. Stopping emotional eating requires activating feel-good feelings in the here and now, and appreciating what you already have. Comparing your current body to what it used to be, or to someone else's, diminishes your power to do that. When you catch yourself comparing your body image to someone else's or longing for what used to be, find something to appreciate in your life now.

"When I turned to HeartMath to overcome my eating disorders, I had been told that if I did not get my bulimia under control I could die because of the damage it was doing to my body. I would binge eat everything in the fridge late at night and get sick the next morning, then go to the store and do it again! Finally, as I caught my ghostly face in the bathroom mirror one morning after a binge, I realized I had hit rock bottom. I did not want to die. I got a piece of paper and a pen, and wrote a contract with myself which I actually signed and dated, in which I promised not to eat between the hours of 8:00pm and 5:00am (my vulnerable binging time). I made a commitment to myself that I would use HeartMath tools during that time, instead of eating. I had read somewhere that a NASA study showed it only takes 21 days to create a new habit, and break an addiction, so I wrote into the contract that I would do this for 21 days. Somehow having a discreet amount of time I was committed to, made it less daunting and more manageable, than if it was perceived as a lifelong sentence and struggle.

My addiction to food, which came out of post traumatic stress from living in a war zone, was so strong that I could not fall asleep at night without eating several boxes of crackers or the equivalent in some other carbohydrates. So I ended up staying up all night some nights in order to stick to my contract, just breathing in through the heart to get through the night. It took a lot of grunt work at first, a lot of heart power, to stick to it. Uncomfortable feelings that I had been using food to suppress showed up. I used the Notice and Ease tool late into the night, to allow the tears and even withdrawal symptoms like itching and heat to come and go without rushing to get rid of their sensation with eating. I found with Notice and Ease I could release the discomfort if I sat with it long enough, without reaching for food. After a week I started to feel better, and to have more energy during the day in spite of the disruption to my sleep. It got easier and I started relating better to the people in my life, and performing better at school, too.

Until day 18. This was the real test of my HeartMath tools. Something happened at work that worried me deeply, and I caved in that night and had some cookies after 8:00pm. I was devastated. I felt that I had totally let myself down, and would have to go back and start the whole thing all over again. I was crushed. It was the hardest thing to face emotionally, to let myself down like that. But it was also the most important moment in the journey. My heart, as I used Notice and Ease with my sense of failure, would not allow me to maintain that "all or nothing" attitude. It had forgiveness and care for me, and appreciation for all that I had done in the 18 days I had stayed committed. This was powerful, and different from my normal reaction. Normally, because I had a few cookies, I would have fallen off the wagon completely and eaten everything in the cupboard. Instead, my heart had me go to bed breathing forgiveness and appreciation for myself. It was as if that had been the missing link all along, and a more valuable thing to experience than sticking to it all "perfectly". Allowing myself to be "imperfect" without punishment was freeing in ways I could not have imagined. Much to my surprise, when I woke up the next day my food cravings were gone. Gone! In only 18 days (not even 21!). And I can honestly say they have not come back in over 10 years! A lifelong struggle with food had ended in less than three weeks once I was able to forgive and love myself. Thanks to HeartMath. Eating disorders, whether anorexia, bulimia or obesity often have stress at their root. We starve, overeat or binge eat in reaction to unresolved emotional issues. Eating disorders can be a way to narcotize feelings you do not know how to identify, transform, and respond to in a different way. Using the HeartMath technology and the intuitive intelligence of the heart can help you identify the messages your feelings are delivering, discern which feelings are accurate and which are coming from emotional memory or "old survival software," and respond to what you feel with clarity."

**Sheva Carr, CEO of Fyera and Project Coordinator
of the Stopping Emotional Eating Beta Test**

Part 2
The *HeartMath Stress and Weight Management Program*

There are five steps in this Program.

The first step *is to identify your stress triggers and stressful emotions that propel stress-related eating and weight gain.*

The second step *is to learn two simple HeartMath tools, Notice and Ease™ and the Power of Neutral to reduce emotional stress and help stop emotional eating.*

The third step *is to build internal coherence with the Quick Coherence® Technique and HeartMath technology to start changing your emotional diet, help sustain your commitments and make behavior changes you want to make.*

The fourth step *is learning the Freeze Frame® and Attitude Breathing™ Techniques to take the drama out of emotional challenges, connect more deeply with your heart's power and intelligence, make attitude shifts and to find new perspectives.*

The fifth step *is learning to make the exciting change from emotional eating to intuitive eating, using the Freeze Frame Technique with the HeartMath device to listen to your heart's intuitive discernment on what, when and how much to eat.*

These steps are progressive. To get the most out of this Program, you'll want to answer the self-study questions, learn and practice the tools provided in each section. This Program is designed to empower you to instate new behaviors and habits. Go as fast or as slow as you'd like, but stay steady with your practice for six weeks. If you slip up, have compassion for yourself, and jump right back in where you left off. After you finish the Program, it's important to keep using the tools, techniques and HeartMath technology for maintenance—to manage stress and to reach and maintain your optimal weight.

So let's get started.

Step 1
Identify Your Stress Triggers and Stressful Emotions

First, it is important to identify the sources of stress that may be contributing to emotional eating and weight gain. As you well know, not all stress is the same. Stress and emotional disturbance can make it difficult to stay on any diet. Some events may create stress that sets off stress eating for you and others may not, so it's important to understand the stress triggers that provoke your emotional eating.

For example, an argument may be stressful at first, but once it is resolved from the heart, you may end up feeling more at peace than before it happened. Rushing to meet a deadline can be stressful, but you may find the challenge exhilarating. Comforting a friend through a difficult time may be stressful, but leave you feeling closer and more loving. None of these stressors may trigger the desire to eat or go off your diet, because they resolved into a positive attitude and satisfying feeling.

Positive feelings make you feel more content with your life and therefore more likely to stick to your diet. Positive emotions revitalize and renew. But some positive feelings also need balancing. Joy or over-excitement can cause an emotional energy swing where you throw care to the wind and "reward" yourself with high calorie food then feel stressed about it later.

The important thing is to recognize which kinds of situations and issues are triggers for you. Your closest friend may feel very nervous every time she has to give a speech, but you may love giving speeches. Your partner may feel uneasy about throwing a party, but you may love entertaining.

On the other hand, you may feel inexplicable anxiety about a vacation in a new locale or asking for a raise. Our emotional triggers are often as unique as our personalities. But there is undoubtedly a pattern to the kind of issues that make you prone to reach for food. Knowing what they are gives you leverage.

What's Your Kind of Stress that Provokes Emotional Eating?

Take a minute and evaluate what propels you to reach for food to comfort yourself.

Your Stress Eating Assessment

Which of these areas are likely to provoke stress and emotional eating in you?

Personal stress
- ☐ Self-image
- ☐ Self-judgment and guilt
- ☐ Relationships
- ☐ Health
- ☐ Work
- ☐ Not enough time
- ☐ Other_____

Family stress
- ☐ Lack of connection
- ☐ Communication issues
- ☐ Too many expectations
- ☐ Judgments and blame
- ☐ Other_____

Friends or Associates stress
- ☐ Communication issues
- ☐ Too many expectations
- ☐ Loneliness
- ☐ Boredom
- ☐ Other_____

Job stress
- ☐ Difficult boss and/or co workers
- ☐ Unrealistic expectations
- ☐ Perfectionism
- ☐ Feelings of overwhelm (deadlines, priorities, overload, etc.)
- ☐ Lack of control
- ☐ Judgments and blame
- ☐ Other_____

What else triggers stressful feelings that result in emotional eating for you?

_____

_____

_____

Stress and Emotions

At the core, all stress is emotional stress because it affects how people feel. Whether you experience it as mental, emotional or physical stress, if you unmask the word stress it's about how you feel inside. Stress is registered in your feelings as tension, strain, pain, overwhelm, anxiety, frustration, angst, depression or disturbing undercurrents that you can't find a name for but still sap your energy and leave you feeling washed out. As these undercurrents occupy your thoughts and feelings, they make it hard to stay with your commitments. We all experience these stressful feelings or attitudes from time to time. It's important to identify the ones you experience often. The following is a list of feelings and attitudes that create stress. Circle the ones that you experience a lot of the time.

- Angry
- Bored
- Lonely
- Deprived
- Impatient
- Irritated
- Frustrated
- Worried
- Anxious

- Depressed
- Insecure
- Perfectionism
- Being Judgmental
- Resistance
- Rebellion
- Guilt
- Blame
- Fear
- Other_____

Now ask yourself how often you feel these attitudes and feelings during a day or a week? What do you do when you feel them? Do you try to shove them aside? Do you brood over them? Do you judge or blame others or yourself? Fill in the following worksheet to get a clear picture.

Stressful emotion or attitude	How often?	What do you do?

Now ask yourself *how often* you experience positive attitudes and feelings, such as love, appreciation or gratitude, genuine care or kindness, compassion for yourself or others, forgiveness of yourself or others, joy or peace during a day or a week? What do you do when you feel these positive emotions? Do you enjoy or savor them? Do you cut them off or deny them? Do you get over-stimulated by them and reward yourself with eating? Do you direct them into creative actions? Fill in the following worksheet to get a clearer picture of your emotional landscape.

Positive emotion or attitude	How often?	What do you do?

Consider the situations, conversations, and events, you've encountered over the past few days. How much time did you spend in stressful emotions that drained your energy and how much time did you spend in positive emotions that revitalized your energy? When you allow stressful emotions and attitudes to dominate your day, or try to cover up your feelings, it becomes difficult-to-impossible to change your eating habits. No matter how good your intentions are, stressful emotions build up inside you and create emotional weight.

Emotional Weight

A lot of weight that people carry around is subconscious emotional weight fueled by unresolved emotional issues, lack of self-worth and underlying insecurity. The accumulation of emotional weight negates your power to lose physical weight because it saps the energy you need to sustain discipline. You try, but then go back to old eating habits and the weight that's familiar—where you subconsciously feel comfortable. The body is designed to want to revert to what's familiar. If feeling bad is familiar to you, then in an odd way you may feel more comfortable feeling bad—until you instate a new pattern.

For example, once insecurity sets in, it's such a strong emotion that it causes a drain on your emotional energy reserves, which causes a drop in the effective functioning of your biochemistry and metabolism, which then creates the urge to go off your diet plan. After you do that, you feel more insecure. This is because emotions, biochemistry and your nervous system are all linked together.

Your body's metabolic set point can get reset from stress eating over time. The part of your brain that signals to you that you're hungry doesn't discriminate whether your body is hungry or your emotions are hungry. It just knows you are hungry. So you crave food. The reverse can occur with anorexia. Emotional stress can shut down the brain's hunger signals, even when the body needs nourishment.

Stressful emotions, disgruntled emotional undercurrents and insecurities all release cortisol and other stress hormones into your system that actually tell your body to go into survival mode. Too much cortisol ultimately causes a redistribution of fat to the waist and hips, even though you may be eating fewer calories. In fact, many people gain weight *when they aren't overeating,* due to increased cortisol levels from stress. Releasing stressful emotions is an inside job, yet the tendency is to try and do it from the outside, through burying yourself in work or projects or through habits, like emotional eating.

Emotional eating offers a biochemical band-aid effect. It changes how you feel for awhile, but it doesn't deal with the cause of your stress. Emotional issues have to be dealt with from the inside or they will run a continuous biochemical loop, causing you to continue what you don't want to do—continuously eat or be obsessed about eating or do "yo-yo" dieting.

One of the most common emotional eating patterns is "yo-yo" dieting. Losing a little and gaining it back, and then dieting some more, then gaining it back. When we bypass what's going on emotionally inside, we often end up in "yo-yo" dieting. Yo-yo dieting usually follows emotional ups and downs, which just puts further strain on the emotions and body. When we are accustomed to looking outside ourselves for stimulation or comfort or for the next quick fix diet, we aren't looking to see what's really happening inside. But the power of your heart can help change this.

Step 2
Reduce Emotional Stress

You have identified the stressful feelings that can trigger emotional eating for you. Now the next step of this Program is to reduce emotional stress by learning two simple tools that enable you to:

1. identify your stress triggers that cause emotional eating as they come up;
2. redirect your emotional energy;
3. increase inner security by re-aligning your heart, mind and emotions.

As you use the two tools, *Notice and Ease* and the *Power of Neutral,* you build new strength to shed emotional build up that can contribute to physical weight. Through activating your heart intelligence and changing your emotional diet (the feelings you feed inside), you can change your biochemistry and build a healthy self-security and self-esteem.

For accelerated results, start learning and using HeartMath technology if you haven't done so already and then focus on deepening your use of the device in Weeks 3 and 4.

Many people are in denial of or simply unaware of their stress triggers or stress reactions as they are occurring. They may become aware after the fact—after their energy drains, or after a miscommunication, or after physical aches and pains develop, or after they've unconsciously subdued the emotion through stress eating. It's important to learn to acknowledge and *treat* (but not with food) stressful emotions as they come up. These two tools are designed to help you do this.

Tool #1 - *Notice and Ease*

Notice and Ease is a simple yet effective tool for acknowledging emotions. You can learn to release many stressful feelings and stop their energy drain by doing the following simple steps.

1. Notice and admit what you are feeling
2. Try to name the feeling
3. Tell yourself to e-a-s-e - as you gently focus in your heart, relax as you breathe, and e-a-s-e the stressful feeling out.

Practice the *Notice and Ease* tool at least 10 times a day at home, at work, talking on the phone, driving in the car, standing in the line at the store, and so on, just to learn to acknowledge whatever you are feeling. At first you might not be able to name the feeling. You may think you are feeling nothing. Ask yourself, "Is there tension anywhere in my body?" Ask yourself, "Have I been worrying about anything that may have left a residue in my feelings?" Ask yourself, "Am I feeling peaceful and at ease?" Whatever you are feeling, try to give it a name, acknowledge that you're feeling it, and then add ease to the feeling in step 3.

Appreciate yourself whenever you can identify and admit what you are feeling. Your feelings aren't bad; they are signals that provide you with information. Stressed or over-stimulated feelings are signals that something is out of balance. Once you acknowledge and accept what you are really feeling, that helps you befriend the feeling, which takes some of the intensity or resistance out of the emotion. As you gently focus in your heart area, relax as you breathe, and ease the stress out. This starts to bring your system back to balance.

As soon as you have thoughts about food or feel the desire to eat something, use the *Notice and Ease* tool. See if there is an underlying feeling of anxiety, sadness, loneliness or even a vague insecurity feeding those thoughts or urges. You'll start to distinguish the difference between craving foods to cover up these feelings and real hunger.

Tip—Always use the *Notice and Ease* tool right before you start eating a meal and even while you are eating, to help bring more balance to what you choose to eat and how much you eat.
 After you have practiced the *Notice and Ease* tool 10 times a day in the above ways for three days, then add Tool #2, *Power of Neutral.*

Tool #2 – *Power of Neutral*
The next HeartMath tool to learn is a simple yet powerful approach for neutralizing and discharging stressful emotions. It's called the *Power of Neutral.* It teaches you to use the power of your heart to bring your mind, emotions and physiology into a more neutral state. Think of Neutral as a "time-out zone" where you can step back, neutralize your emotions, and make better decisions.

Here are the steps of the Neutral tool:

1. Take a time out, breathe slowly and deeply. Imagine the air entering and leaving through the heart area or the center of your chest.
2. Neutralize the stressful thoughts and feelings as you continue to breathe.

Try to disengage from your stressful thoughts and feelings as you continue to breathe.
Continue until you have neutralized the emotional charge.

After you use the *Notice and Ease* tool, and admitted what you are feeling, if you were unable to ease the stress out, use *Neutral* to help align your heart, mind and emotions to neutralize the stressful feeling. An important facet of neutral is the awareness that there may be more to a situation you are reacting to than what you currently know. Neutral is an attitude of openness to reserve judgment and wait to react until you have more information. You take a time-out by choosing to step back from the stress feeling and release the emotional significance you are placing on the issue. Step 1 helps draw the energy out of your head, where negative thoughts and feelings get amplified. Just breathe slowly and deeply in a casual way as you imagine the air entering and leaving through the center of your chest and heart area. In step 2, just having the intent to neutralize the stressful thoughts and feelings, as you continue to breathe through the heart, can help you release a lot of the emotional energy and neutralize the emotional charge.

Using Neutral doesn't mean that your frustration, worry or other stressful feeling will have totally evaporated. It just means that the charged energy has been taken out and you have stopped the stress accumulation. Even if you can't totally neutralize the stressful feeling, just the effort to shift into neutral will give you a chance to regroup your energies and refocus. As you practice Neutral you will build your power to tell intrusive disturbing thoughts and feelings, "Thanks for stopping by, but I'm not going to feed you," and mean it. This will start to change your emotional diet – the feelings and thoughts you keep feeding yourself. You will begin to see more clearly what triggers your emotional eating habit and you'll build power to neutralize the emotional drive fueling your habit.

Practicing Neutral also helps to "rewire" the metabolic pattern of overeating in your physiology. Even if you don't feel a difference right away, making a sincere attempt to apply the steps of Neutral helps to balance your nervous system and hormones in ways that can reduce cravings and gradually allow your body to better metabolize food. As your metabolism and cravings change, this makes it easier to neutralize emotional stress. You start to feel better about yourself and a positive feedback loop is created whereby emotional management reinforces a physiological change, and the physiological change makes it easier to neutralize stress. Each time you go to *Neutral,* you are taking an important step to reprogram both your emotional and physical habit patterns. It helps to remember that it won't always be as difficult to go to *Neutral* as it can seem in the beginning; as you establish new neural habits, it gets easier and easier!

Practice the *Neutral* tool at least 10 times a day for four days to really get to know this tool. Sometimes you may feel you have to use *Power of Neutral* 20 times or more a day. That's fine, because you are developing the power to manage your emotional triggers and repatterning the physical imbalances that cause cravings with this tool.

Practice Plan:

- Use the *Notice and Ease* tool at least 10 times a day for the next three days.
- Then add *Power of Neutral* at least 10 times a day for four days.
- Memorize the *Notice and Ease* tool and the *Power of Neutral* steps. Use these two tools until you know them by heart before you go onto the third step of this Program.

Step 3
Increasing Heart Coherence with Heart Rhythm Technology

The next step in this Program is to monitor your heart rhythms and coherence level to establish a new baseline of coherence in your mental, emotional and physical systems over the next two weeks. To do this, you use your device with the *Quick Coherence* Technique. Using the device, you will be able to:

a) See the level of coherence in your heart rhythms – low, medium or high.
b) Use the *Quick Coherence* Technique to improve your coherence level.
c) Improve your coherence baseline to reset your stress response and attitude.

The HeartMath device measures your heart rhythm pattern (or heart rate variability– a key to self-regulation) and it measures your coherence level. It lets you know when your heart rhythms have moved into a more coherent pattern. When there is coherence in your heart rhythms, your entire body gets more in sync. As you increase your coherence level, your nervous, cardiovascular, hormonal, metabolic and immune systems work together more efficiently and harmoniously. This helps to reset your desire to eat when you aren't hungry and to offset the effects that stress eating has had on your physiology. You may also notice a reduction in physical stress symptoms.

Through daily practice with your device, you will raise your *coherence baseline*. This means that you will have more heart rhythm coherence occurring naturally within your system throughout a day. This gives you more ability to manage your emotions and stop emotional eating. It also helps you sustain positive feelings and attitudes longer and have more intuitive discernment.

When you first start using your technology, you will probably be in low coherence which is normal. As you practice coherence-building techniques, like the Quick *Coherence* Technique, your coherence level will improve.

The heart coherence technology will help you relieve emotional stress the more you use it. It is not a magic quick fix, but it will help you accumulate coherence energy, so you stay more emotionally balanced through the flow of life. Using the device gives you more leverage to cushion and deflect the things that would normally cause stress and disruption. It also helps you recoup more quickly from things that have stressed you out. As you practice with the device, you will increase your baseline of coherence (the amount of coherence that naturally occurs in your system when you aren't using any tool) and this helps to reset your stress response.

There is a learning curve at the beginning, while you are adjusting to this new way to take responsibility for your emotions and attitudes. It may seem a little unusual at first to turn to a heart technology, instead of food, for emotional self-care. Stick with it! This may be one of the most important things you ever learn to do.

It's your heart coherence that makes it easier to sustain emotional commitment, reduce stress and create healthier eating habits. The technology will help you increase your heart coherence and heart power.

"I am now convinced that dieting does not work in most cases of overweight. The real problem is emotional overeating. I gave a lecture in Avignon last June at a symposium (350 psychiatrists) on emotions and overeating, and since then, have been overwhelmed with propositions for lectures, speeches and teaching.

Since I have started using the HeartMath device with overweight patients, I no longer give any dietary or nutritional information whatsoever. And yet my patients have the best results in weight loss I've seen in all my years of practice. People are losing weight just by increasing their heart coherence and with no prescribed diet at all.

People know what they should eat. They can find that information. It's only the emotional side of eating that stops them from eating what they should. Once they increase their heart coherence, eating in a way that's balanced and beneficial for them comes naturally."

David O'Hare, M.D.

Dr. O'Hare is a psychiatrist with a specialty in Nutrition and Obesity for over forty years. In France, he is the practitioner with the most extensive experience using HeartMath's technology for weight loss. He sees 10–12 patients a day, most of whom are overweight.

"I struggled with dieting my whole life. Both my parents were obese, and I remember being self-conscious about it and putting myself on my first restricted diet when I was just four years old. By the time I was 16, I was a professional ballet dancer and so obsessed with remaining thin to look good on stage that I once went three weeks without eating anything but a muffin, while rehearsing eight hours per day. It took its toll for sure. I would have unexplained emotional outbursts, my menstrual cycle stopped and I broke an ankle with a stress fracture due to bone density loss.

At age 27, I had a heart attack, which doctors attributed to the loss of muscle mass in my heart from starvation. But I would absolutely panic at the thought of gaining weight. After my heart attack, my metabolism had slowed so severely and I was under so much stress, that I began to pack on pounds no matter how little I ate. I went into a phase of binging and purging, eating out the entire refrigerator at night (probably from being so depleted for so long), and then feeling so bloated and sick the next day that I would fast for a couple of days, then start the whole cycle over again. I could not find balance and my body, my school work and my mind were paying a high price. It was a nightmare. And then I found HeartMath.

Shortly after my heart attack, I got an emWave® device from one of my doctors. It was amazing. I never thought there could be a real cure for anorexia, but for me the emWave device was it. I would get on the emWave feeling fat and ugly, and after getting into coherence I could see my body more clearly and appreciate it. I started to feel good about how I looked, and to just plain feel good for the first time ever.

Four weeks exactly after I started using the HeartMath technology device I got my period for the first time in six years. So I guess my hormones starting balancing right away. The HeartMath technology device taught me how to eat in a balanced way. If I was starving myself, I could see right away the effect that it was having on my heart rhythm (not good) and sometimes with just a small snack I could bring myself into coherence. Conversely, if I went into a panic and was tempted to binge, I would get on the HeartMath technology device first, and that would invariably calm me down and the cravings would subside.

I still like to spend a minute or two on the HeartMath technology before I eat anything, because it is like a mirror for whether my body really needs food, or if I am eating emotionally. I don't mind the little bit of time that it takes, because the pay-off in how I feel is tremendous. My metabolism has gone back to normal, and I eat full fabulous meals (even chocolate and desert!). I am in better shape than when I starved myself, I can think more clearly, and my body is stronger than ever before. I am so grateful to have found the emWave and hope that other people find the benefit from it as well."

"Preferred to remain anonymous"

Tool #3—Quick Coherence Technique

1. Focus your attention in the area of the heart. Imagine your breath is flowing in and out of your heart or chest area, breathing a little slower and deeper than usual.

Suggestion: Inhale 5 seconds, exhale 5 seconds (or whatever rhythm is comfortable)

Putting your attention around the heart area helps you center and get coherent.

2. Make a sincere attempt to experience a regenerative feeling such as appreciation or care for someone or something in your life.
   Suggestion: Try to re-experience the feeling you have for someone you love, a pet, a special place, an accomplishment, etc., or focus on a feeling of calm or ease.

You can learn more about this simple technique in several ways:

1. Read about the *Quick Coherence* Technique in the Inner Balance app Quick Start Guide or in the HeartMath tab on your iOS device.
2. If you have an emWave 2, use the Coherence Coach® that is on the software (it's already installed in the emWave Pro) to learn the technique.

As you practice the *Quick Coherence* Technique and the other tools with your HeartMath technology, you create a coherent alignment that invites or draws in more of your spirit and higher discernment faculties—your intuition. This creates a cushion between you and stressors that come up so they don't drain you as much, and provides you with more clarity on how to respond.

Heart Feeling:

Step 2 helps you increase coherence on the HeartMath device without having to remain as conscious of your breathing rhythm. If it was hard for you to find a positive or regenerative feeling or attitude, take a moment now to remember a couple of times when you felt calm, joyous or uplifting feelings. Write those experiences down or memorize them so they will be easy to recall the feeling when you practice the *Quick Coherence* technique.

Don't worry if you also feel some discomfort while you're breathing in a positive or regenerative feeling or attitude. Even a little heart feeling starts to clear subconscious emotional patterns. Just befriend any discomfort with compassion and ease. Building a new baseline of coherence is an unfolding process. Just keep up a *genuine* heart intention to hold the attitude of appreciation or care, (love, compassion or forgiveness) as you practice the *Quick Coherence* Technique.

3—Practice the Quick Coherence Technique while using your HeartMath Technology.

Once you have learned the technique, you are ready to use it along with your device. Your goal in using the *Quick Coherence* Technique with the technology is to get the red light on your emWave (red dot on your Inner Balance Trainer) to turn from red (low coherence) which is normal, to blue (medium coherence) which is much improved, to green (high coherence) which is the optimal state.

1. Focus your attention in the area of the heart. Imagine your breath is flowing in and out of your heart or chest area, breathing a little slower and deeper than usual.
    Suggestion: Inhale 5 seconds, exhale 5 seconds (or whatever rhythm is comfortable)

Putting your attention around the heart area helps you center and get coherent.

2. Make a sincere attempt to experience a regenerative feeling such as appreciation or care for someone or something in your life.

Suggestion: Try to re-experience the feeling you have for someone you love, a pet, a special place, an accomplishment, etc., or focus on a feeling of calm or ease.

Watch the light (or dot) change from red to blue to green. Sustain blue or green as long as you can. Make it a gentle process and continue to feel appreciation or care.

If you practice the technique with your eyes closed, which can be helpful when you are first learning, you'll be able to tell when you have shifted into medium or high coherence through listening to the change in audio tones if you have the sound turned on.

The more you practice the *Quick Coherence* Technique with the HeartMath technology, the easier it gets to move from low coherence, into medium coherence and then into high coherence—the optimal state where your heart, brain and nervous system are in sync. Observe what thoughts or feelings take you out of medium or high coherence, then use the *Quick Coherence* Technique to go deeper in the heart and shift back into coherence. This develops emotional flexibility and resilience.

Practice increasing your coherence ratio (percentage of time you are in high coherence vs. medium coherence vs. low coherence). When you can stay in high coherence at challenge level 1 for long periods, move to challenge level 2. On days you feel more stressed or when it's hard to stay in high coherence, go back to challenge level 1 to help reset your system. Getting "in the green" at challenge level 1 is always beneficial and will have a carryover effect.

Use your HeartMath technology at least four times a day: in the morning when you first get up and before you decide what to eat for breakfast, before lunch, before dinner and before you reach for a snack anytime. You can also use the HeartMath technology with

Power of Neutral or the Freeze Frame Technique or the Attitude Breathing Technique to get into coherence before potentially stressful situations, or to recoup more quickly after a stressful experience, or before bed for a more restful sleep.

If you find you aren't able to shift back into coherence easily, using the breath pacer can help you re-enter the coherence state. However, it takes feeling genuine heartfelt attitudes to sustain coherence. The technology's breath pacer is "smart" in that once you get into high coherence (green light), the pacer will adjust its speed to help you stay "in the green." Sometimes people go into very shallow breathing when trying to activate a positive feeling. If this is your tendency, just breathe a little more deeply while generating a feeling of appreciation, gratitude, love or care and you'll move into higher coherence more easily.

The more you see the real-time feedback on the HeartMath device, the more it motivates you to improve your coherence skills. But don't expect perfection from yourself as you use the device. That only adds stress! Instead appreciate the progress you are making. By giving you immediate feedback, the device can eliminate any doubt that you are making progress.

Everyone goes through different energetic rhythms during a day, a week or a month, so there will be times when it can be harder to "stay in the green" or harder to maintain positive feelings and focus. At these times, breathe the heart feeling of compassion for yourself and non-judgment in Step 3 of the Quick Coherence Technique. Just staying in as much coherence as you can during each session will establish a more balanced rhythm between your mind, heart and emotions, while increasing your coherence baseline over time.

It's important to have balanced expectations of yourself while you practice weight management. Your goal is not perfection, but progress. Give yourself credit for your daily successes. Appreciation is a jump starter that adds coherent energy to help sustain your practices and make the changes your want to make. Appreciate when you manage your attitudes and emotions. Appreciate when you use the device and the other tools, and when you have compassion and nonjudgment toward yourself. Appreciate when you make better choices on what to eat or when to exercise.

Some people enjoy tracking their progress. You can do so on your device. Don't fall into the trap of feeding your inner critic by scrutinizing or judging yourself—the most important thing is to feel good while using your device and that will motivate you to use it more! Make it a fun game.

Practice Plan—

- Use the *Quick Coherence* Technique with your device to get into coherence at least four times each day: Before breakfast, before lunch, before dinner, before you reach for a snack.
- Other important times to use your device: Before potentially stressful situations, to recoup more quickly after a stressful experience, before bed for a more restful sleep.
- Use your device for five minutes or more each time. Once a week, do a 10 minute or longer session with your HeartMath technology.
- Practice increasing your *coherence ratio* (the percentage of time you are in high coherence vs. medium coherence vs. low coherence).
- Continue to use the *Notice and Ease* tool and the *Power of Neutral* as needed as you move through your day.

More Tips On Using Your HeartMath Technology

- Make a commitment to use the device for three to five minutes *before* you act on a craving or a binge. You can always go back to whatever you were going to eat afterwards, but sometimes just giving yourself a three minute time out on the device can rebalance your system and put you in touch with what your body and belly really want and need. Using the device this way gives you heart power where will power will not work.

- Use the device *after* you have fallen off the wagon into old habits to find self-forgiveness and to get back on track. Instead of using the cookies you ate as a justification to go for ice cream too, hook up the device and get back on track!
- Using the device to prepare for a meeting helps activate a deeper clarity, mentally and emotionally, while increasing your capacity for intuitive listening and speaking from the heart. This gives more substance and effectiveness to your communications.
- When you feel time deprived, anxious or overloaded during the day, use the device to help restore drained emotional "accumulators". The human system accumulates or drains energy depending on how you respond emotionally to the events of your life.

Use the device whenever you want to center yourself and be more in the present. The HeartMath technology helps this process by letting you know when you're really present. Each moment you spend in the present (rather than ruminating about the past or projecting about the future) saves and accumulates energy.

Step 4
Changing Your Emotional Diet

The fourth step in this Program is to learn a powerful technique, called the *Freeze Frame* Technique. The *Freeze Frame* practice will help you to:

a) take the drama and significance out of emotional reactions.

b) refocus your emotional energy and shift your emotional state to align with your core heart values.

c) connect with your heart intelligence and intuitive discernment.

How Do You Eat Emotionally?

Identify some of the main characteristics of your emotional eating habits. Below are some common emotional eating patterns. Think back over the last week and the last month to see which ones apply to you. See if you can identify what feelings triggered the pattern and write them down.

Eating Pattern	Emotional Trigger
You ate when you weren't hungry	Loneliness? Boredom? Insecurity? Other?
You skipped meals and binged on snacks	Frustration? Overload? Other?
You went on an eating splurge	Relationship stress? Disappointment? Other?
You kept a hidden stash of food	Insecurity? Rebellious? Other?
You sneaked food when no one was around	Tension? Embarrassment? Other?
You did "yo-yo" dieting	Felt imbalanced? Stress got to you? Other?

List other emotional eating patterns or other emotional triggers that you have that are not on this list:

_____

_____

_____

_____

Now, write down any new insights you've gained from this exercise.

_____

_____

_____

_____

Next, list your favorite comfort foods. What types of feelings do eating comfort foods bring you? Right before eating them? While eating them? After eating them?

Comfort foods I eat the most   *Feelings they give me*

_____   _____

_____   _____

_____   _____

_____   _____

Other things that give me these feelings (e.g. taking a bath, going for a walk, stretching, talking to a friend)

_____

_____

_____

_____

Can you see how these feelings are heart feelings? Experiment with practicing the *Quick Coherence* Technique, and using your device to generate these feelings without the food or other activities that help you feel them.

Part of the problem with emotional eating is the speed at which it occurs. Often we aren't conscious of emotional eating or stress eating until after the fact. In five minutes we may have emptied a bag of crackers and chowed down 1,200 calories without realizing it. When we don't balance our emotions and moods in the moment, we compensate by eating snacks or comfort foods without regard to their calorie content or healthfulness, and then often feel guilty afterwards.

When we feel stressed or time crunched, we grab fast foods we know aren't good for us. Sometimes, we could buy something healthier just as fast, but we don't. It doesn't seem as appealing. We subconsciously choose foods that alter our brain chemistry in a way that makes us feel better. Something that increases our blood sugar or releases endorphins into our brain gives us respite from the pressures or stresses we feel, even if it's temporary.

Not living up to our own expectations can become an obsession that consumes a lot of our thoughts, feelings and energy. Then the emotional diet we are feeding ourselves is full of self-judgment, self-blame, guilt, despair and shame, all of which drain our energy and make us want to comfort ourselves with pie or cake or other foods.

It's important that we acknowledge, neutralize and release the negative emotions and attitudes that we feed ourselves. It's equally important that we learn how to refocus our emotional energy and shift our emotional state to comfort ourselves from inside-out. Using the list of other activities and behaviors that bring comfort as replacements for seeking comfort in food can also help, especially while you are learning to the *Freeze Frame* Technique and activate positive feelings from your own heart first.

The *Freeze Frame* Technique will help you change your emotional diet to include more positive feelings and attitudes, and then help you connect with your heart intelligence and intuitive discernment.

The *Freeze Frame* Technique builds on the *Power of Neutral,* the *Notice and Ease* tool and the *Quick Coherence* Technique, by connecting you with the intelligence of your heart and higher brain. Noticing what you feel, easing it out through the heart, getting neutral, and then adding positive emotion with the *Quick Coherence* Technique all prep your physiology to clear static so you can hear your intuition. With the *Freeze Frame* Technique you can tap into your intuitive intelligence to select a better emotional diet and make better food choices. It is like "freezing the frame" on your internal camera so you can see your thoughts and feelings more clearly, then activating the core values of your heart to expand your lens of perception. This brings in new heart feelings and intuitive intelligence, which we call heart intelligence.

Have you ever felt so upset that you had to close the door to your office or bedroom or go for a walk to clear your head? You do these things so you can take a step back from the situation, calm down, regroup and find a new strategy or solution. The *Freeze Frame* Technique helps you do all this quickly, within a few minutes, on the spot wherever you are.

Tool #4—*Freeze Frame* Technique

1. Acknowledge the problem or issue and any attitudes or feelings about it.
2. Focus your attention in the area of the heart. Imagine your breath is flowing in and out of your heart or chest area, breathing a little slower and deeper than usual. *Suggestion: Inhale 5 seconds, exhale 5 seconds (or whatever rhythm is comfortable).*
3. Make a sincere attempt to experience a regenerative feeling such as appreciation or care for someone or something in your life.
4. From this more objective place, ask yourself what would be a more efficient or effective attitude, action or solution.
5. Quietly observe any subtle changes in perceptions, attitudes or feelings. Commit to sustaining beneficial attitude shifts and acting on new insights.

Here's why this technique works.

Learning to "*Freeze Frame*" in the heat of the moment or after a stressful situation can save tremendous amounts of energy and prevent the consequences of emotionally charged reactions, whether stress eating or saying something that you later regret.

The *Freeze Frame* Technique helps take drama and significance out of your reactions to a situation. By taking the drama out, your wise self can talk things through with your confused or stressed self, and save you a lot of problems. That wise self is your heart intelligence.

Some of the steps are similar to the techniques you've been practicing. It can be helpful to understand the physiological changes that occur. The simple act of focusing on your heart combined with a deeper level of breathing draws energy away from stressful thoughts and feelings. It interrupts the body's stress response, and also starts to bring more order into your heart's rhythms. Psycho-physiologists know that as your heart's rhythmic beating pattern becomes smoother and more ordered, then it's easier to experience a positive feeling and attitude. Ordered heart rhythms and positive attitudes also make it easier to gain intuitive clarity.

The third step is to make a sincere effort to connect with the core values of your heart and activate a regenerative feeling, like appreciation, care, compassion or kindness. Positive feelings and attitudes increase the *coherence* in your heart rhythms and the signals your heart sends to your brain. While still focusing on breathing through your heart area, you now want to 'feel' a positive feeling. One of the easiest ways to do this is to remember someone, some place or something that feels good to you and that you appreciate. Examples could be a wonderful vacation, a fun time at a sports event, or the appreciation or love you feel for a close friend, family member or a pet. It could even be recalling the feeling that comes while eating your favorite comfort food. The important thing is to feel it, not just think it. You want to relive the moment and sustain that positive feeling for 20 seconds or more.

Notice what you experience. How do you feel after doing this step? Any stressful feelings or thoughts you had should at least be diminished.

If your emotional reaction has been so strong you had difficulty finding a positive feeling, have a genuine "I mean business" attitude to take the significance or the big deal out of the situation and really move negative emotions into a more neutral state. Even after you have made an attitude shift, there can still be emotional residue left. That's normal. Just take the significance out of it, stay in neutral and appreciate yourself and the efforts you are making. If you hold a non-judgmental, appreciative or forgiving attitude toward yourself and others who are involved, the emotional residue often releases.

Practicing steps two and three of the *Freeze Frame* Technique increases synchronization and coherence between your heart, brain and emotions, which facilitates higher cognitive functions that normally are compromised during stress. Coherence is a psycho-physiological state that aligns your heart, emotions, mind, body and spirit. Your ability to think clearly and objectively is enhanced so that you can view the issue, interaction or decision that had been stressing you from a broader more balanced perspective. Coherence is a state very similar to what people call a state of "presence" or "the flow" and athletes call "the zone."

Now in step four you can ask yourself what would be a more efficient or effective attitude, action or solution that would balance and de-stress your system. If you listen, your intuitive heart intelligence may bring you new insights and discernment.

Step five helps you listen to your heart's intelligence. Keep your focus on your heart area and quietly sense any shifts in perception, attitude or feelings. These changes can be subtle. Don't go looking for them with your intellect. Stay open to sensing them from your feelings and intuition. The ordered messages the heart is now sending to the brain can result in thoughts, attitudes or feelings that give you better discernment. You may have intuitive feelings about what to eat and what not to eat. Note any changes in perception, feeling or attitude that you experience once you do the *Freeze Frame* steps.

Commit to any new perceptions or solutions—then act on them as soon as you can. You may want to write them down to help you remember. If a new attitude or perception starts to waiver, this is a normal occurrence. Gently bring it back to awareness and recommit until it is anchored.

Through practice of the *Freeze Frame* Technique, sensing the changes in perceptions, attitudes and feelings will become quicker and easier for you. What's most important is that you have reversed the impact that negative or stressful attitudes and feelings were having on your system just a few moments before and brought more order and coherence into your system.

Tool #5—Attitude Breathing Technique

With strong emotional reactions, it also helps to add what we call the *Attitude Breathing* Technique at this point. You admit the feeling or attitude that you want to change, such as anger, anxiety, blame, sadness, self-judgment, frustration, guilt, feeling overwhelmed, etc., and then breathe a replacement attitude. You do this by selecting a positive attitude and then breathing the feeling of that new attitude in slowly and casually through your heart area. For example, if you are worried, breathe calm; but remember—this requires breathing the attitude of calm until you actually *feel more calm*. When you feel more calm, that's when you have made the *energetic shift*. Keep breathing the feeling of the new attitude to make it more real.

Next are examples of replacement attitudes. As you breathe these replacement attitudes, tell yourself to take the significance and drama out of the situation or resistance you feel. Tell yourself, "Take the significance out." Repeat this to yourself as you breathe in the new attitude.

Unwanted attitudes	Replacement attitudes
Feeling stress	Breathe neutral to chill out
Feeling anxiety	Breathe calm and balance
Feeling overwhelmed	Breathe ease and peace
Feeling sadness	Breathe appreciation and compassion
Feeling blame or guilt	Breathe compassion and nonjudgment

Use the attitude replacement list above and note which replacement attitudes feel the best to you. You can also look at the list you created of feelings your favorite comfort foods give you, and experiment with breathing those feelings as replacement attitudes. Breathe that feeling of comfort in through the heart, and out through the heart. What do you notice? What happens to your body? Your emotions? Your mental clarity?

As you practice the *Attitude Breathing* Technique, stay open to new replacement attitudes from your heart intuition. Being able to access feelings of comfort without food, even for just a moment, is a big step toward being free from emotional eating. A moment to shift is all you need, and that's good news because sometimes a moment is all you have.

As you continue using the *Attitude Breathing* process, the increased coherence in your heart's rhythm reaches the brain's cognitive and emotional centers to reinforce the positive feeling or attitude shift you have made. You can practice the *Attitude Breathing* Technique at any time to help you make an emotional shift and then sustain it. This increasingly creates an inner comfort and ease that helps release the craving for outer comfort or food.

Practice Plan—

- Practice the *Freeze Frame* Technique at least three times a day for the next week and learn the steps by heart.

- Use the *Freeze Frame* steps after strong emotional disturbances to refocus your emotional energy, shift your emotional state, and connect with your heart intelligence and intuitive discernment.
- Use the *Attitude Breathing* Technique to help sustain emotional shifts.
- Keep a written journal, if you choose, of any insights you gain from using the *Freeze Frame* Technique
- Continue to use the *Notice and Ease* tool or *Power of Neutral* several times a day as well.

Use this Practice Plan until you feel solid with it, then move onto Step 5: learning to make the exciting change from emotional eating to intuitive eating, using the *Freeze Frame* Technique to follow your heart's intuitive discernment on what, when and how much to eat.

"I've struggled since I started modeling at age 13 and had to always focus on how I looked. The stress of being turned away from jobs because I wasn't thin enough took a toll on me. If I was a size 6, maybe I could be a 4. If I was a 4, maybe I could be a 2.

I struggled with overeating at times, then restrictive diets and exercising like crazy. It's been a battle gaining then losing between 5 lbs and 30 lbs. for years. When things got overwhelming, I'd inevitably put on a little weight, and then struggle to lose it again for work. I never felt fulfilled in myself. I needed to find balance and that's when I found HeartMath.

Coming to my heart and using the tools to find out what my deeper truth is and reminding myself of that makes all the difference. Watching and witnessing if I'm really in my heart, wanting to reset my body's rhythms, helped me choose healthier food and not overeat.

When you listen to your heart, your body's appetite kind of takes care of itself and you don't have to be the food police. Of course it takes practice to get there. It doesn't just happen overnight.

In the past I have gotten to the 'right' weight many times. But it was from being focused on this exercise program and this diet, and I gave myself no room to live. I felt I couldn't express myself under these rigid conditions, so I'd eventually fall off.

Once you reach your weight goal and stay there by going to your heart and practicing that regularly, then it's less about making big changes and more about learning to tune to your heart to live in a more balanced way all the time.

When I started to practice HeartMath tools, little by little I witnessed myself making different choices. I noticed when I took a few minutes to be proactive to go back to the heart and use a tool, it would kind of take care of things before situations escalated to where I would want to use food or overeat to compensate. Taking that time for me to get more connected with my heart each morning eventually carried over into to the days that I didn't take that time in the morning. I could see the play out of increased coherence, in that I still didn't want to eat more."

Rhonda Willoughby, fashion model, Los Angeles, California

Step 5
Making the Exciting Change from Emotional Eating to Intuitive Eating

As you practice these techniques and use the HeartMath device you will begin to develop a new sensitivity to yourself. You'll increasingly recognize the stress triggers and feelings that have led to stress eating and be able to regulate them more. You'll shift to more positive and balanced emotional states and increase coherence in your system. Most importantly, you'll start to find a more balanced approach to eating, from the inside-out.

Through following Steps 1–4 of this program, you have been activating the intelligence and coherent power of your heart. This enables you to change your eating patterns and use intuitive discernment on what and when to eat. Heart intelligence unfolds practical intuition – the ability to intuitively discern a better course of action in the moment. Increasing coherence in your heart rhythms helps make that intuitive information more available to you.

Research has shown that intuitive information is registered first in the heart which then transmits the signal to the brain/mind. As you build a new coherence baseline with the HeartMath techniques and technology you use, you create more coherent alignment between your emotions, mind and body which is the foundation for accessing more intuitive discernment.

The following exercise helps you increase intuitive discernment and apply it to your food choices.

Intuitive Eating Exercise

In this exercise you will use a slightly modified version of the *Freeze Frame* Technique with your device before you decide what to eat for breakfast, lunch and dinner, and especially before you reach for a snack. It's helpful to do this exercise within a half hour before you eat.

Turn on your device and get into medium or high coherence. While in coherence use the *Freeze Frame* Technique in this adapted version.

1. Take a time out so that you can temporarily disengage from your thoughts and feelings—especially stressful ones.
2. Shift your focus to the area around your heart. Now, feel your breath coming in through your heart and out through your heart. *Practice this for 10 seconds or longer.*
3. Make a sincere effort to activate a positive feeling. *This can be a genuine feeling of appreciation or care for someone, some place or some thing in your life*
4. Ask yourself what would be an efficient, effective attitude to hold as you decide what to eat.
5. Quietly sense any shifts in perceptions, attitudes or feelings.
6. Listen to what your heart intelligence (your intuitive discernment) tells you to eat (or not eat).

As you practice this exercise, your intuitive heart intelligence will guide you increasingly on what to eat, when to eat and how much to eat. As you develop intuitive sensitivity to your body, you will choose foods that are more beneficial for you. A bonus: you will also find your intuitive discernment increasing in other areas of your life. To get the most benefit from this Intuitive Eating exercise, practice it daily for two weeks or more. You may want to write down insights you have each time you do the exercise to help you remember to apply them. If your heart guides you to go on a specific food plan, that's fine. Just keep using the *HeartMath Stress and Weight Management Program* and your heart power to carry out your intentions. Don't be afraid to make changes along the way guided by your heart's intuitive discernment. Appreciate the intuitive discernment you are developing in other areas of your life as well.

"Your intuitive heart is the GPS for finding the shortest and most effective route between intention and its destination."

– Doc Childre

Many people who practice the *Freeze Frame* Technique begin to experience their heart like an intuitive guidance system that helps them know what to eat, what diets to follow, what relationships to nurture and what exercise is right for them. What is best for one person might not be best for another.

We live in a world where there are as many diets as there are dieters. With so many weight loss programs to choose from (some of which even contradict one another), it makes a huge difference to have an inner guidance system that helps you to discern what's best for you. Your heart intelligence is tapped into what your body needs. As you learn to listen to and follow your heart's guidance, you can more easily find a course of action that is suited to your unique needs and that changes as your needs change.

"Before I found HeartMath, dieting was a constant prison guard keeping me from feeling at ease in social situations and family functions. I wanted to take care of myself, but I also did not want to be a burden on my family and friends. My desire to stick perfectly to my diet, and at the same time be the perfect guest, made dinner parties an absolute nightmare. I tried to avoid them at all costs, so I would not have to make my special requests for low fat low carb meals and be the only one skipping the wine and the dessert. Since working with the Freeze Frame Technique, I have learned to follow my heart's intuition in social situations, knowing where I can share a little bit here or there in what everyone else is having, without feeling like I've blown it completely. Freeze Frame practice has also made me feel less self conscious when asking for dressing to be put on the side, or other little tricks that allow me to be in a social situation while maintaining my weight loss goal. The balance and confidence the Freeze Frame Technique has given me to have everything in moderation—even my diet regime—has led me to a place inside where I can trust myself. The heart has been a key freeing me from

the jail cell of my own making, where I imprisoned myself with formulas and regimens and beat myself up if I didn't stick to them, which would make me want to hide and eat even more. As a result of trusting my heart's guidance, I have had both a physical weight loss, as well as a major emotional weight loss in my friendships and relationships too. I am so grateful for the heart's intuitive knowing."

Sheva Carr, CEO of Fyera and Project Coordinator of the Stopping Emotional Eating Beta Test

Practice Plan

- Use the modified version of the *Freeze Frame* Technique with your device within a half hour before each meal or snack to help you discern what to eat and how much to eat.
- Practice this Intuitive Eating Exercise for the next two weeks to develop your intuitive discernment skills and make the exciting change from emotional eating to intuitive eating.
- Write down insights you have along the way to help you remember and apply them.
- Continue to use the *Notice and Ease tool, Power of Neutral* and the *Quick Coherence or Attitude Breathing* Techniques as you move through your day to keep developing your stress management skills.
- Appreciate the intuitive discernment you are developing and applying in other areas of your life as well.

"I was so humiliated when my doctor wrote "obese" on my chart. I felt, 'That's not me; that's not who I am.' But I was in denial. I weighed over 200 pounds. It was on a trip to Paris with some friends when I finally realized, 'I'm really unhappy, unhappier than I've ever been.' I tried so hard not to get my photo taken on the trip. I couldn't stand

to look in the mirror and see the double chin and flabby arms. I didn't want to see me that way in a photo either. I knew I had to lose 50 to 75 pounds. A friend of mine kept telling me I had will power, but I kept getting angry with her and told her, 'You don't look like this if you have will power.'

When I signed up for HeartMath at my weight loss clinic, I had tears in my eyes because I didn't believe this would work. I followed the Program along with exercise for a week and lost 6 lbs. I took it step by step. I paralleled my experience to an alcoholic. It was one temptation at a time. I would ask myself, 'Am I hungry, or what is this pull to eat about?'

I have found that a lot of what it was about was emotion. Food has been a silent comforting friend – it never judged me, didn't talk back and was always available. I used the HeartMath tools and discovered my heart is more of a friend. I'm now a size 6, down from 16W-18W. Now when I feel the pull to food, I can think of HeartMath tools and stop myself and ask do I really want to? And I don't. That's heart power not will power. I'm more conscious now because I want to, not because I have to. If I choose to have a cookie now, it's fine, because I choose to do it. It's balanced from my heart."

S.M., Salinas, California

Summary

You've learned how to use your HeartMath technology along with tools and techniques that you are applying to manage and transform stress and stop emotional eating. As you practice the *HeartMath Stress and Weight Management Program,* you will feel the benefits—not only in weight and appearance, but in other aspects of your life.

You'll start seeing results within a short period of time. It usually takes at least six weeks to change a habit, so make a commitment to study and use the HeartMath Stress and Weight Management Program for at least six weeks. Make it a fun learning process. Look at it as an adventure that will build lasting benefits for you.

You can take control of your stress and your emotions with the HeartMath tools, techniques and technology. You can change your emotional diet as part of a wholeness diet as you follow the Program.

Here is a summary of the HeartMath Stress and Weight Management Program:

Week 1

1) Identify the sources of stress that may be contributing to your emotional eating habits. Tracking your stress signals and stress reactions helps to pinpoint where you need to manage and release stress.
2) Learn and practice the tool *Power of Neutral* at least 10 times a day and take a time out to neutralize stress reactions. Just the effort to shift into neutral will give you a chance to regroup your energies and build your power to manage emotional triggers.

Part 3
Study Guide

This program is a caring investment in yourself—the most important investment you can make. We encourage you to follow the instructions as they are given and genuinely learn to use the simple tools provided. You can feel better and do better in all areas of your life – and lose weight at the same time.

1—Learn to Operate your HeartMath technology
Free video tutorials are available on the HeartMath technology products at www.heartmath.com.

2—Take a 1 hour Telephone Class
Learn to use your HeartMath technology with free phone-based product training at www.heartmath.com.

3—Schedule Time to Commit to Your Six-Week Program and Yourself
* 10–15 minutes every morning or evening
* 3–5 minutes before each meal and before bed
* 1 hour per week for reading, doing the program exercises and writing in your journal (if you choose).

Take a moment now to enter these times in your calendar for six weeks and make a non-negotiable commitment to yourself to treat this time as you would an important business or health care appointment.

4—Establish Your Team
Consider how you learn best. Are you a solo study that learns best on your own? Or a social learner who needs interaction with others to stay motivated?

Set yourself up for success, and put the pieces in place that will help you achieve your desired goal to stop emotional eating.

HeartMath® Certified Coach/Mentors are available to coach you through your Six-Week Program. Visit www. heartmath.com.

Quick Start: Tool Cheat Sheet

Notice and Ease tool:

1. Notice and admit what you are feeling.
2. Try to name the feeling.
3. Tell yourself to e-a-s-e, as you gently focus in your heart, relax as you breathe and e-a-s-e the stressful feeling out.

Power of Neutral:

1. Take a time out, breathe slowly and deeply. Imagine the air entering and leaving through the heart area or the center of your chest.
2. Neutralize the stressful thoughts and feelings as you continue to breathe.

Try to disengage from your stressful thoughts and feelings as you continue to breathe.

Continue until you have neutralized the emotional charge.

Quick Coherence Technique:

1. Focus your attention in the area of the heart. Imagine your breath is flowing in and out of your heart or chest area, breathing a little slower and deeper than usual.
   Suggestion: Inhale 5 seconds, exhale 5 seconds (or whatever rhythm is comfortable)
   Putting your attention around the heart area helps you center and get coherent.
2. Make a sincere attempt to experience a regenerative feeling such as appreciation or care for someone or something in your life.

Suggestion: Try to re-experience the feeling you have for someone you love, a pet, a special place, an accomplishment, etc., or focus on a feeling of calm or ease.

Freeze Frame Technique:

1. Acknowledge the problem or issue and any attitudes or feelings about it.
2. *Focus your attention in the area of the heart. Imagine your breath is flowing in and out of your heart or chest area, breathing a little slower and deeper than usual. Suggestion: Inhale 5 seconds, exhale 5 seconds (or whatever rhythm is comfortable).*
3. Make a sincere attempt to experience a regenerative feeling such as appreciation or care for someone or something in your life.
4. From this more objective place, ask yourself what would be a more efficient or effective attitude, action or solution.
5. Quietly observe any subtle changes in perceptions, attitudes or feelings. Commit to sustaining beneficial attitude shifts and acting on new insights.

Attitude Breathing Technique:

1. Admit the feeling or attitude that you want to change, such as anger, anxiety, blame, sadness, self-judgment, boredom, frustration, guilt, feeling overwhelmed, etc.
2. Breathe a replacement attitude (make a list). You do this by selecting a positive attitude and then breathing the feeling of that new attitude in slowly and casually through your heart area. For example, if you are worried, breathe calm. This requires breathing the attitude of calm until you actually feel more calmed. That's when you have made the energetic shift.

3. Keep breathing the feeling of the new attitude to make it more real.

Intuitive Eating:

After you have learned and practiced the other tools and are able to stay in coherence on the HeartMath technology device for a few minutes, you will be ready to start practicing this tool. Use this slightly modified version of the *Freeze Frame* Technique with your HeartMath technology device before you plan a meal or decide what to eat for breakfast, lunch and dinner, and before you reach for a snack. It's helpful to do this exercise within a half hour before you eat.

1. Start your HeartMath technology and get into medium or high coherence. While in coherence use the *Freeze Frame* Technique in this adapted version.
2. Take a time out so that you can temporarily disengage from your thoughts and feelings—especially stressful ones.
3. Shift your focus to the area around your heart. Now, feel your breath coming in through your heart and out through your heart. Practice this for 10 seconds or longer.
4. Make a sincere effort to activate a positive feeling. This can be a genuine feeling of appreciation or care for someone, some place or some thing in your life.
5. Ask yourself what would be an efficient, effective attitude to hold as you decide what to eat. Quietly sense any shifts in perceptions, attitudes or feelings.
6. Listen to what your heart intelligence (your intuitive discernment) tells you to eat or not eat.

What are the differences between the tools?

The tools are similar but there are subtle differences, which you will discover as you practice them. It's fun to learn which one's work best for you in different situations. If you find a favorite tool, it's fine to use that one more often. If you get emotionally stuck, try one of the other tools.

Notice and Ease and *Power of Neutral:*
Often we overeat in reaction to emotions that we are not consciously aware of. The *Notice and Ease* tool helps you identify what you are feeling, so that you can take charge of it. The *Notice and Ease* tool is designed to make you more aware of what your automatic or reactive feelings are. Neutral, on the other hand, helps you to disengage from a strong emotion once you identify it, so that you can reclaim the energy the emotion is sapping from your system by consciously neutralizing its charge instead of adding drama.

Neutral is one of many attitudes you can use as a replacement for charged or stressful emotions that cause emotional eating. Neutral is a stepping off point to shifting to a positive attitude. Neutral is, in fact, a necessary step before being able to use the *Freeze Frame* Technique and gain new perceptions and insights.

Notice and Ease allows you to become aware of attitudes and emotions that are draining your energy and triggering overeating. Overeating is in and of itself often an attempt to feel differently, or to generate a different attitude.

Quick Coherence:
The Quick *Coherence* Technique helps you activate feelings that produce a physiological state called "coherence". Coherence produces an ordered pattern in your heart's rhythm that turns the light on your HeartMath technology first to blue and then green. The *Quick Coherence* Technique is designed to be used with the HeartMath technology to help you get into an optimal state for resetting your body's emotional and metabolic responses, and building a new baseline of coherence.

Freeze Frame and *Attitude Breathing:*

Many people think that feelings "just happen" to them. With these power tools, you can begin to consciously choose new feelings, thereby changing your behaviors, responses and outcomes in life.

Attitude Breathing helps you to apply replacement attitudes that are more effective for your health, well being, and eating habits. The *Attitude Breathing* Technique supports you to find comfort and attitude adjustments from the heart, without food. Use the *Attitude Breathing* Technique:

a) when it is hard to find a positive or regenerative feeling.

b) to build a list of replacement attitudes that work for you.

c) to anchor and reinforce attitude changes your heart intuition guides you to in the *Freeze Frame* Technique.

10–15 Minute Daily Practice Plan

The accumulation of emotional weight negates our power to lose physical weight because it saps the energy we need to maintain discipline and enjoy life. This 10–15 Minute Daily Practice Plan is designed to empower you to recharge your own energy, to refuel without food and plug the emotional energy drains that might cause you to reach for food for emotional comfort.

If you spend 10–15 minutes on this daily practice plan, you will develop the inner resources to respond to stress triggers with the power and perspective of your heart's intelligence, instead of with overeating. As emotional weight lifts, so will your physical weight. You can use this plan to jump start your progress in this six week program and to sustain your results once you've completed the program.

1) Identify stressors that trigger your emotional eating.
   A good way to do this is to make a list at the end of each day of events, interactions with people, activities and even

inner attitudes that left you feeling out of sorts or that you reacted to by eating emotionally. This is your energy deficit list. Your deficits will begin to turn into assets (and you'll have more energy) as you use the tools in the program. Awareness of what sets off your emotional eating is step one.

2) Identify assets you are building. Make a list at the end of each day of events, interactions with people, activities and even inner attitudes that left you feeling energized and happy. This is your gratitude or energy asset list. Appreciation adds fuel to your system (without food) and opens up higher brain and perception centers to look at things that trigger your stress eating with new eyes.

3) Spend five minutes hooked up to your device, appreciating the things on your gratitude list as you anchor in the "green." Even if you can find one thing to appreciate each day, it will make a big difference.

4) Turn your attention back to your stress triggers, or deficit list. Use the *Neutral and Notice and Ease* tools and the *Freeze Frame* Technique, to take the drama out of stressful situations, ease their emotional impact out through the heart and receive guidance from the heart on more efficient responses. See if you can find a benefit to each deficit, turning it into something you can appreciate and add to your asset list. If you cannot do that, you can at least neutralize the emotional drain and minimize the cravings created.

5) During the day, set an alarm to go off hourly on your phone or watch or an egg timer, or make notes in your computer calendar to remind you to practice the *Quick Coherence* Technique, *Notice and Ease*, *Neutral* or the *Attitude Breathing* Technique several times during the day to stay balanced in the heart.

Summary

You've learned how to use your HeartMath technology along with tools and techniques that you are applying to manage and transform stress and stop emotional eating. As you practice the HeartMath Stress and Weight Management Program, you can feel the benefits—not only in weight and appearance, but in other aspects of your life.

You'll start seeing results within a short period of time. It usually takes at least six weeks to change a habit, so make a commitment to study and use the HeartMath Stress and Weight Management Program for at least six weeks. Make it a fun learning process. Look at it as an adventure that will build lasting benefits for you.

You can take control of your stress and your emotions with the HeartMath tools, techniques and technology. You can change your emotional diet as part of a wholeness diet as you follow the Program.

Physician networks in the USA, France and Mexico have sent us stories of their clients using the HeartMath techniques and technology to lose weight and keep it off. They all say that once people regulate their attitudes and stop emotional eating, the weight loss follows. The HeartMath technology then helps them to emotionally and physically integrate back into a normal diet – without regaining the weight they lost.

Murray, a corporate lawyer, had high blood pressure with obesity. He was extremely unhappy and stressed out. He knew everything he should be doing, but he couldn't stick to it. He thought he was in control at work, but didn't think he could control what he ate. After learning how to get into heart rhythm coherence with the HeartMath technology, Murray realized that it wasn't food management he needed, but heart management. Instead of letting the time pressures on his job make him anxious, he found a way to stay calm. When there was a stack of phone messages on his desk and his Inbox was overflowing, he used his heart to take it in stride. At the end of the day, instead of bringing all the stresses of work home with him, he was able to shift attitude, leave it at the office and enjoy his time with his family.

Before learning about HeartMath tools and technologies, the only thing Murray knew was to feel overwhelmed. He was in such a demanding job that everybody said it was "understandable" that he was stressed out, but no one offered any solutions for finding balance. After all, it's commonplace for attorneys to be stressed out. With Murray's blood pressure levels, it was well on the way to costing him his life.

When he learned about HeartMath, he practiced diligently. After twelve weeks he looked like a different person. "It's spooky how different I feel," Murray said. He'd dropped nearly 30 pounds. His blood pressure had gone from 162/110 to 122/84. He was far better able to deal with stress. And to his great satisfaction, he no longer had an urge for emotional eating.

Additional Resources

While you are practicing the *HeartMath Stress and Weight Management Program*, you may want to use other HeartMath resources designed to help you with unresolved emotional issues, including the books *Transforming Anger, Transforming Anxiety, Transforming Stress, Transforming Depression* and *Heart Intelligence: Connecting with the Intuitive Guidance of the Heart*.

If you want personal coaching with the *HeartMath Stress and Weight Management Program*, there are certified HeartMath practitioners and coaches, called HeartMath Coach/Mentors, who are ready to assist you and many health professionals who use the HeartMath tools and technologies in their practices. You can call 1–800-450–9111 or go to www.heartmathproviders.com to find a Coach/Mentor who can work with you in person or over the phone.

I am a Registered Nutritionist. For years now I have been between 10 and 50 pounds above my ideal weight. With my special weird diets, grueling exercise and long history of failing, I wasn't much of an example of a nutritionist. This became my secret painful truth.

Finally, with HeartMath technology, I found the secret missing ingredient: my emotions! Every situation that caused me to reach for food showed up on the HeartMath technology as a messy jagged mess. I was emotionally out of whack!

Using the HeartMath technology, I have lost 15 pounds in the last 2 months and feel great. I have discovered that coherence is essential—especially when I am shopping for food, eating that food and resisting the triggers like TV commercials, smells of baking, the sight of chocolate and dealing with difficult situations and people.

Now when I shift into coherence using the HeartMath technology, my heart rhythm pattern becomes smooth and ordered, and so do my food choices. Thanks!

Karen O'Dwyer, Nutritionist, Toronto, Canada

Appendix

The scientific background behind the HeartMath technology.

Practice with your HeartMath device helps you self-regulate your autonomic nervous system which controls 90% of your body's involuntary functions, including immune system response, hormonal response, metabolic response, digestion, elimination and more. The autonomic nervous system has two branches. One branch is the sympathetic branch that speeds things up. It is activated when you are stimulated or aroused, and speeds up heart rate. The other is the parasympathetic branch, which slows things down. It is activated as you relax and clam down and slows heart rate. The activity in your autonomic nervous system tells the body's organs and glands how to respond. Your sympathetic nervous system gets activated when you are under stress to prepare your body to react to threats, real or imagined. Chronic stress, frustration, anxiety, depression and social isolation are associated with an overactive sympathetic nervous system. The chronic activation of the sympathetic nervous system due to negative emotional states depletes your energy reserves and increases the risk of stress-related health problems. It is also implicated in stress hormone related weight gain and obesity.

Heart rate variability (HRV), a measure of the naturally occurring beat-to-beat changes in heart rate, provides an indicator of heart-brain interactions and autonomic nervous system function. HRV is also highly reflective of stress and emotions and is used to assess people's overall vitality. Emotions especially trigger changes in the autonomic nervous system and the hormonal system.

Changes in the *pattern* of your heart rate (or heart rhythm) are most reflective of your current emotional state. Changes in heart rhythm pattern are independent of heart rate. You can have a coherent or incoherent pattern at high or low heart rates, as the graph below shows. This is a graph of a person feeling frustration, then using the

Freeze Frame Technique to shift into a feeling of appreciation and heart rhythm coherence. You can see that her heart rate stayed between 60 and 90 beats per minute the entire time. *For more information, you can read *The Coherent Heart* e-booklet or view the published studies, available at www. heartmath.org

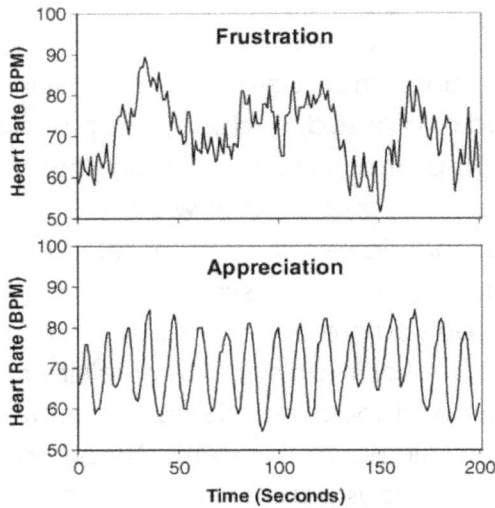

Figure 1. Emotions are reflected in heart rhythm patterns. The heart rhythm pattern shown in the top graph, characterized by its erratic, irregular pattern (incoherence), is typical of negative or stressful feelings such as anxiety, worry, frustration or anger. The jagged and irregular rhythm reflects disorder and disharmony in the ANS, as if the parasympathetic and sympathetic branches of the ANS were fighting each other. This taxes the nervous system and organs, impeding the synchronization and flow of information throughout the body. The bottom graph shows the smooth and ordered heart rhythm pattern (coherence) that is typically observed when an individual is experiencing sincere positive emotions, such as love, appreciation or compassion. The smooth coherent rhythm reflects an ordered synchronization between the sympathetic and parasympathetic branches of the autonomic nervous system.

Over time, if your autonomic nervous system stays disordered, you can experience ongoing stress symptoms, like digestive and metabolic problems, hormonal and immune system imbalances, heart problems, or the onset of chronic diseases like high blood pressure, Type 2 diabetes and obesity. Learning how to regulate your autonomic nervous system and get into heart rhythm coherence and can give you more ability to change your stress reactions and improve your health. It's important to understand that coherence is different than relaxation, as illustrated in the graph on the next page.

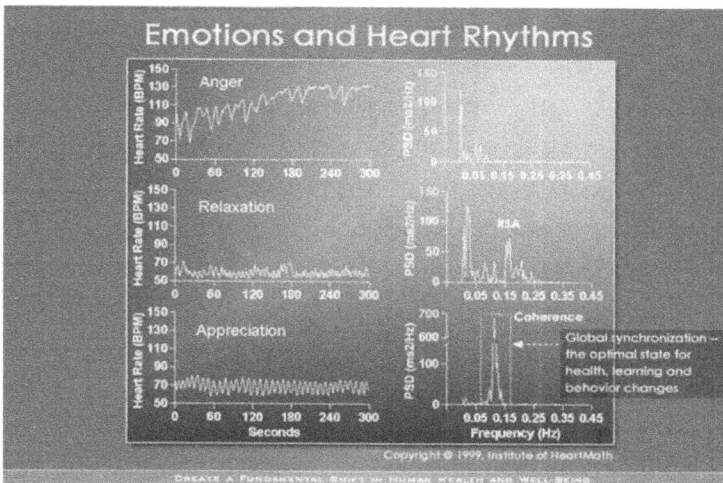

Figure 2. Coherence is different from relaxation. It's feeling relaxed and revitalized at the same time. The top graph shows a typical incoherent heart rhythm pattern for the feeling of anger on the left and the power spectrum for anger on the right. You can see the activity of the sympathetic nervous system (high peak at the left), the parasympathetic nervous system (tiny peak at the right), and the activity in what's called the heart-brain communication loop (tiny peak in the middle).

The middle graph shows a typical heart rhythm pattern and power spectrum for relaxation, with more parasympathetic activity.

The relaxation response will lower heart rate, but it won't create coherence or synchronization between the parasympathetic and sympathetic nervous systems.

The bottom graph shows a typical heart rhythm coherence pattern, generated by appreciation (and other positive emotions). The power spectrum shows one large, narrow peak, around 0.1 Hz, which indicates synchronization between the sympathetic and parasympathetic nervous systems and in the communication between the heart and brain. (Coherence also facilitates cortical functions while incoherence inhibits cortical function.)

Now look at the topmost number on the vertical scale in each power spectrum graph, which indicates the amount of power. In the spectra for both anger and relaxation, the largest peak measures under 150. In contrast, the peak for appreciation (coherence) measures 700! *Synchronization and coherence generate more than five times the power!* Coherence adds power to help you self-regulate emotions and behaviors that aren't serving you, so you can improve your health.

Heart Rate Variability and Impulse Control

In a research study of self-regulation by Dr. Suzanne Segerstrom, published in *Psychological Science*, March 2007 and summarized in a Reuters article entitled "Heart Rate Variability Mirrors Self-Discipline," Dr. Segerstrom describes Heart Rate Variability as "the capacity of the heart to be sensitive and responsive to changing demands, and can indicate our self-regulatory strength."

She suggests that will power is a lot like muscle strength. While some people seem to have more innate capacity for self-regulation, we can all take steps to boost our power.

Heart Rate Variability in Weight Management

Obesity and weight management present many challenges and difficulties for health professionals. As the director of a non-drug biofeedback stress management center at a major teaching hospital, I was always open to new treatment modalities. I particularly wanted treatments that engaged the client actively in their own care and on a daily basis.

As a psycho-physiologist I had spent many years utilizing breathing techniques, heart rate variability, and EEG biofeedback/neurofeedback training for anxiety and panic attacks. Heart rate variability was of interest to me as an undergraduate student early in the 1970's. The pulse itself has been historically monitored by ancient cultures including the Greeks and Chinese for centuries. They were keenly aware of its relationship to health and its diagnostic value. I continued to investigate heart rate variability as a biofeedback technique but found it frustrating because of the lack of good economical equipment for the office setting. Even with the advent of computers little was available for the office based practice.

As an early adopter of the HeartMath technologies I became very comfortable with its unique ability to produce excellent feedback information for myself and the client. Using the technology allows me an in-depth look at a client's emotional physiology and how well they regulate their emotions. I very quickly found myself working with problems such as high blood pressure and irritable bowel syndrome, in a more effective fashion. The device was very effective at helping clients control panic attack and anxiety. It also helps people create an excellent alpha brain wave state that helps clients relax and participate more effectively in their therapy. I was particularly pleased with it in helping ADD/ADHD with children and adults.

In 2003 I created the Institute of Weight Management and Health dedicating my work to weight management and health related weight problems. Although I use many interventions to help individuals manage weight, including food management, lifestyle changes and exercise, the emotional component of over-eating is still the most important issue. Why do people turn to food for relief from the stress in their lives? Until an individual can control the driving forces that cause them to turn to food for relief, they cannot successfully control their weight problem or their life.

The considerations of time, cost and success rate are extremely important to weight management practitioners and clients. The need to change the mostly negative attitudes to positive feelings is also important. The HeartMath technology provided exactly what was needed to deal with the overwhelming negative emotional issues that weight management clients deal with on a daily basis. Instead of endless hours of therapy that may rehash unpleasant negative emotions, the client is trained to move to a positive place in their emotional life. Change the negative attitudes to positive attitudes and the client will lose weight.

Our program includes twelve one hour sessions—twice a month for six months. About half of each session is devoted to heart rate variability training. Our success rate has been greatly increased by adding the heart rate variability training. Although the positive health affects of weight reduction can be immediate and dramatic, the improvement in the emotional condition is often more dramatic and life altering. Successfully controlling the internal physiology can be empowering to an individual whose life has been mostly out of control. In its simplest terms the client learns to stare food in the face and walk away. In doing so the client learns to deal with life instead of eating themselves into a protective cocoon and a sugar high.

Spiking glucose can be an enticing rush, however, the inevitable down side and crash can be depressing and frightening. This may explain the addictive nature of the problem and the cravings or binge eating. Along with the eating comes the guilt and shame that crush self-esteem. Having the ability, calmness and focus to face the truth and deal with it, requires self-control and self-regulation. The HeartMath technologies provide an easy interactive way to involve the client in their own care and their own destiny. Clients often report enjoying the practice time at work and home. Many clients report that their practice time is the only time they get to control themselves away from the influence of external pressures such as work or family. Some clients have described their new found feelings as a clearer sense of self. Some say it has a spiritual nature.

At this time in my practice, it would be fair to say that the HeartMath technology is the main tool I use for most feedback. I would not want to do weight management work without the ability to calm and focus the client. The HeartMath technology's simplicity and ease of use make it client and practitioner friendly. The HeartMath technology makes my practice so much more simple and effective and I could not be more pleased.

Dr. Philip A. Pappas

Dr. Pappas is the program director of The Abington Stress Management Center and The Abington ADD Program. He was formerly the chief operating officer of Abington Behavioral Medicine Associates, a mental health clinic at Abington Memorial Hospital. Dr. Pappas developed Nutritional Health Associates. In 2000, he was appointed director of The Institute of Weight Management and Health. He is author of the book, Irritable Bowel Syndrome—Managing the Problem.

Your Stopping Emotional Eating Companion

emWave® or Inner Balance™

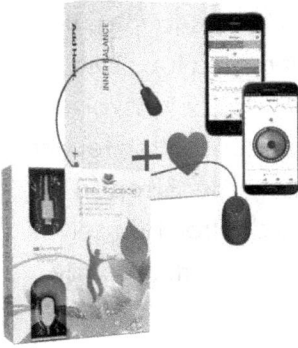

HeartMath's Heart Rate Variability (HRV) technology is a scientifically validated system that trains you into an optimal high performance state in which the heart, brain and nervous system are operating in sync and in balance. We call this state coherence. HeartMath's HRV products measure your coherence level, store your data and connect you to the HeartCloud™ for community support and rewards. As you increase your coherence level, your ability to focus and take charge of emotional reactions improves and you have greater access to your heart's intuitive guidance system for making effective choices.

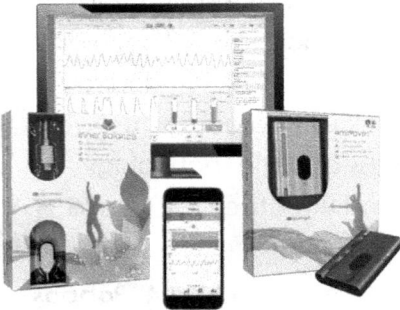

The emWave2® or Inner Balance™

Portable and convenient ways to reduce stress, balance your emotions, increase your cognitive functions and enhance performance. Used just a few minutes a day, this simple-to-use technology helps to transform anger, anxiety or frustration into inner peace, ease and mental clarity. Health, communication and relationships improve.

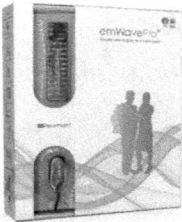

emWave Pro for PC & Mac

Using a pulse sensor plugged into a USB port, emWave Pro collects and translates HRV (heart rate variability) coherence data into user-friendly graphics. It provides a Coherence Coach®, fun visualizers and games that respond to your coherence level. emWave Pro and emWave Pro Plus are multiuser and ideal for classrooms and for health professionals to keep track of client data and progress.

www.heartmath.com or call 1 -800–450-9111

Training and Certification Programs

Add Heart™ Daily Calls
Dial in or log in to join a 10 minute call with a HeartMath staff trainer to increase your mental and emotional fitness and practice the Heart Lock-In® Technique together.

Become an Add Heart™ Facilitator
Become an approved facilitator to learn and share with others some of the science that underpins the HeartMath system, an effective three-step technique for getting into coherence, and how to use the Inner Balance Trainer. In this online course, you learn how to share what you are learning in personal and professional situations.

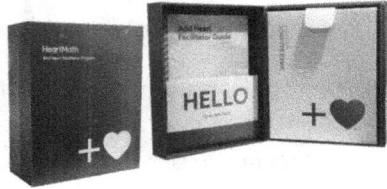

Become a HeartMath® Certified Coach/Mentor
Learn via an 8 week telephone course HeartMath's scientifically–validated tool set and how to teach these tools to clients. HeartMath Coach/Mentors are licensed to teach the HeartMath System in a one-on-one setting.

Become a HeartMath® Certified Trainer
Attend a full immersion 4.5 day certification program. HeartMath Certified Trainers are licensed to provide HeartMath workshops in a 6 hour program, and in shorter modules, or to embed HeartMath modules, techniques, tools and scientific concepts into other training programs.

Become a Licensed HeartMath® Health Professional
The HeartMath Interventions Certification Program includes 6 one hour interactive webinars and video presentations. Health professionals learn how to use HeartMath techniques and technology with patients in various therapeutic and clinical applications.

HeartMath Institute
HeartMath Institute (HMI) is nonprofit organization that researches and develops scientifically based tools to help people bridge the connection between their hearts and minds. It also provides HeartMath programs to social service agencies, and curricula for children and schools pre K-college. **www.heartmath.org**.

Call 1–800-450–9111 or visit www.heartmath.com

Heart Intelligence: Connecting with the Intuitive Guidance of the Heart

By Doc Childre, Howard Martin, Deborah Rozman Ph.D. and Rollin McCraty Ph.D.

Our newest book, Heart Intelligence, provides breakthrough research linking the physical heart to the spiritual (energetic) heart. This book provides simple techniques for accessing our heart's intuitive intelligence for moment-to-moment guidance and discernment

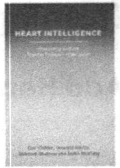

Transforming Depression: The HeartMath® Solution to Feeling Overwhelmed, Sad, and Stressed

by Doc Childre and Deborah Rozman, Ph.D.

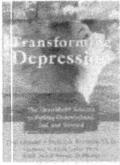

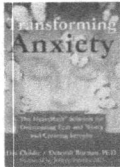

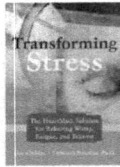

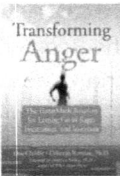

Transforming Anxiety: The HeartMath Solution for Overcoming Fear and Worry and Creating Serenity

by Doc Childre and Deborah Rozman, Ph.D.

Transforming Stress: The HeartMath Solution For Relieving Worry, Fatigue, and Tension

by Doc Childre and Deborah Rozman, Ph.D.

Transforming Anger, The HeartMath Solution for Letting Go of Rage, Frustration and Irritation

by Doc Childre and Deborah Rozman, Ph.D.

The HeartMath Solution

by Doc Childre and Howard Martin

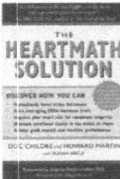

www.heartmath.com or call 1-800-450-9111

HeartMath is a registered trademark of Quantum Intech, Inc.

For all HeartMath trademarks go to www.heartmath.com/trademarks

www.ingramcontent.com/pod-product-compliance
Lightning Source LLC
Chambersburg PA
CBHW060517280326
41933CB00014B/2997